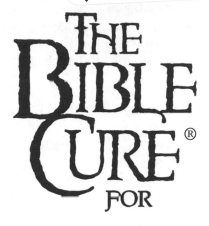

THE BIBLE CURE®

FOR

COLDS, FLU AND SINUS INFECTIONS

DON COLBERT, M.D.

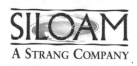

SILOAM

A STRANG COMPANY

The Bible Cure for Colds, Flu and Sinus Infections by Don Colbert, M.D.
Published by Siloam
A Strang Company
600 Rinehart Road
Lake Mary, Florida 32746
www.siloam.com

by the Lockman Foundation. Used by permission.
(www.Lockman.org)

Library of Congress Catalog Card Number:
2003113322
International Standard Book Number: 0-88419-938-X

This book is not intended to provide medical advice
or to take the place of medical advice and treatment
from your personal physician. Readers are advised
to consult their own doctors or other qualified
health professionals regarding the treatment of their
medical problems. Neither the publisher nor the
author takes any responsibility for any possible consequences from any treatment, action or application
of medicine, supplement, herb or preparation to any
person reading or following the information in this
book. If readers are taking prescription medications,
they should consult with their physicians and not
take themselves off of medicines to start supplemen-
tation without the proper supervision of a physician.

05 06 07 08 09 — 98765432
Printed in the United States of America

Stop Suffering!

W e live in a sea of germs. They live in the food we eat, the water we drink, the air we breathe and especially on the hands we shake. In fact, they are present on virtually every surface on this earth. That's why it's impossible not to be exposed to outbreaks of colds and flu.

But have you ever wondered why some people catch more colds and flu than others? The answer lies within the incredible shield of defense God provided to protect your physical health: your body's mysterious and complex immune system.

Your body is God's house, the temple of His Holy Spirit. (See 1 Corinthians 6:19.) God promises to build it up and make it strong with His wisdom and establish good health by providing you with understanding.

That's what this Bible cure is all about. It's packed full of spiritual insight, powerful faith, natural wisdom and sound medical advice—all to help you begin walking in God's divine health.

Massive Attacks

We are under an attack of massive proportions. In the U.S. alone there are an estimated one billion colds every year. Colds usually occur between October and March, and the average adult contracts two to four colds annually while the average child gets six to ten colds a year. It's no wonder that common colds are the leading cause of absenteeism in the U.S., causing about seven lost workdays per person per year.[1] Much of this suffering is completely unnecessary, as you will see. So get ready to reclaim your total health—body, mind and spirit.

Addressing the Spiritual Roots of Disease

Interestingly, as a Christian medical doctor I have studied and prayed about the causes of disease, and increasingly I have discovered that most diseases have very strong spiritual roots. Although traditional medicine often sees the body, mind and spirit as being very separate, in truth they are not. A vital link exists between the spirit, soul and body. That's why this Bible Cure book will also explore the significant link between colds, flu, sinus infections and the spirit. Although you may think such links could not possibly exist when it comes to these very common miseries, what you read in this book may genuinely surprise you.

God's desire is that you walk in total and complete health. This Bible cure is filled with hope and encouragement for understanding how to help your body achieve optimum performance. In this book, you will

uncover God's divine plan of health
for body, soul and spirit,
through modern medicine, good nutrition
and the medicinal power
of Scripture and prayer.

Throughout this book, key Scripture passages will help you focus on the power of God. These divine promises will empower your prayers and redirect your thoughts to line up with God's plan of divine health for you—a plan that includes total victory.

This Bible cure will give you a strategic plan for conquering colds, flu and sinus infections in the following chapters:

If you are tired of suffering with colds, flu and sinus infections, take fresh confidence in the knowledge that God is real, He is alive and He loves you more than you could ever imagine. You *can* enjoy vital health—body, soul and spirit.

It is my prayer that these powerful, godly insights will bring health, wholeness and spiritual refreshing to you. May they deepen your fellowship with God and strengthen your ability to worship and serve Him, fulfilling your divine purpose on the earth.

—DON COLBERT, M.D.

A BIBLE CURE PRAYER
FOR YOU

Father God, thank You for being a great, wise and wonderful Creator. Thank You for providing a powerful shield of defense to protect my body from every enemy and foreign invader. As I read through the pages of this book, open the eyes of my understanding so that I can actively begin to participate in strengthening my body's defense. Reveal to me ways that I may be tearing down my own health and hindering Your healing power. Most of all, Lord, open my heart to understand You in a new and dynamic way as Healer of my body and Lover of my soul. In Jesus' name, amen.

Chapter 1

A Mighty Army

If your eyes were instantly opened to the spiritual realm, you would see realms of angels defending and protecting you and your family from attacks of darkness. God's spiritual army contains forces too numerous to count. The Bible says, "The chariots of God are twenty thousand, even thousands of angels: the Lord is among them, as in Sinai, in the holy place" (Ps. 68:17, KJV).

Nevertheless, God isn't only the Creator of the spiritual realm. He also made the physical realm and everything in it. And the natural realm works in similar fashion to the spiritual one.

In the natural, your body is under constant physical assault. An army of trillions of microscopic germs and organisms—all with the potential of defeating your health—assaults your body every day. Germs and bacteria are everywhere. It's estimated that one trillion bacteria make their residence on the surface of your skin. That's just one person's skin. With such an intense germ warfare assault against your health, is it even possible to enjoy and maintain perfect health?

Absolutely yes! In fact, just as He provided for your defense in the spiritual realm, your Divine Creator also has equipped your body with a physical defense system that is nothing short of marvelous. Your immune system sets up a biological guard with many lines of defense.

Let's take a closer look at the natural guard God has set up to protect and defend your physical health.

Your Amazing Immune System

When functioning at optimal levels, your immune system is completely capable of defending your health against the normal onslaught of germ warfare waged against your body. It is an amazing biological army more powerful and sophisticated than anything else known to mankind.

Think about it; on other continents where the populations have been exposed to many potentially deadly diseases that instantly might do our bodies great harm, the people there respond to these deadly germs as we would respond to a common cold. Why? Their immune systems have encountered these diseases over the years and have learned how to conquer them.

Let's turn now and carefully investigate this amazing army that has been defending your body since shortly after you were born.

Military Strategy

Every military strategy involves a first line of defense. An enemy first encounters resistance to its attack at the first line of defense.

Your immune system also has a first line of defense for your body. When it comes to colds, flu and sinus infections, your immune system's first line of defense is your skin and mucous membranes.

Viruses and bacteria cannot penetrate the skin unless there's an entrance through a cut or break. That's when an inflammatory response occurs, which sends your immune system into high gear in order to rid the body of the bacteria or virus.

Cold and flu viruses enter the body through the mucous membranes, creating inflammation and swelling of the membranes. Swollen, inflamed mucous membranes cause the mucous glands to secrete more mucus as they work to rid the body of the virus. But too much swelling can block off sinus openings so that they cannot drain. Stagnant mucus then becomes infected with bacteria, creating a sinus infection.

Now the immune system marshals troops to launch a second line of attack. The immune system uses scavenger cells, called *phagocytes*, to rush into the area of inflammation and eat or ingest the bacteria.

White blood cells (called *neutrophils*) also are part of this attack plan. These cells circulate in the blood, seeking infection in order to respond. In similar fashion, a second type of cell (called *macrophages*) patrol the tissues seeking and killing bacteria by eating and digesting them. These troops are well known for releasing substances into the bloodstream that cause fever to be produced.

Now, what if the first and second arms of attack have been marshaled and the enemy keeps coming? That's when your immune system calls for special forces.

Employing Special Forces

The body's third line of defense against invading bacteria and viruses is natural killer cells. Natural killer cells exist for no other purpose than to sweep through the bloodstream killing any and every foreign invader in its path, including viruses, bacteria, fungi, parasites and even infected cells and cancer cells. These cells operate like special forces—they work on their own independently of other immune responses.

The body's invaders have been pushed back but not wiped out. The big guns are coming to finish them off.

Bringing in the Big Guns

Those big guns are the T-cells and B-cells, which strategically work in very different ways—like the army and navy—to protect and defend your health from colds, flu and sinus infections.

Let's take a look at these two forces of war that stand ever ready to defend your health.

T-cells

T-cells are deployed throughout the body on a seek-and-destroy mission. They work like heat-seeking missiles as they travel mainly through the lymphatic system as well as the bloodstream. T-cells are matured in your thymus, which is a small gland located above the heart. It is large during childhood but shrinks considerably in adulthood.

This military branch of immunity service fights viruses, yeast, bacteria, fungi and parasites, especially the ones that are present within cells. The three main types of T-cells include:

- Helper T-cells
- Cytotoxic T-cells
- Suppressor T-cells

Helper T-cells sound an alarm that an invader is present. They also assist the stronger cytotoxic T-cells in killing a virus or bacteria. Helper T-cells also send a signal for the macrophages to move in. Many of the other immune cells cannot begin their work without permission from the helper T-cells. Suppressor T-cells, on the other hand, prevent helper T-cells from overreacting and attacking normal cells.

Helper T-cells also tell the B-cells to produce a kind of smart bombs called *antibodies*.

B-cells

Every day your body creates approximately a billion B-cells, which come from bone marrow instead of the thymus and are present in the lymph nodes. B-cells do not circulate in the blood. Instead, their job is to produce antibodies, a substance that neutralizes the effect of a foreign invader.

B-cells produce antibodies against viruses and bacteria with the help of T-cells. Once the antibodies are produced, they are then sent to the bloodstream like smart bombs to lock on to an invader and destroy it. Antibodies attach to bacteria, viruses, parasites, fungi and other microorganisms, and they either damage the microorganisms or mark them so that they can be recognized and destroyed by macrophages.

An Amazing Shield of Defense

The immune system is so sophisticated that it is divinely programmed by supernatural creative genius to defend against all viral and bacterial intruders. Through helper T-cells and B-cells, and through the production of antibodies and cytotoxic T-cells, the immune system actually breaks the codes of various viruses, bacteria and other diseases. It learns how to recognize and attack specific viruses and bacteria. Once it has broken the code of any threat or disease, that particular molecular enemy will lose its edge of power for attack.

Amazingly, your immune system even possesses a memory so that it can rapidly attack bacteria or a virus that is recognized from a past infection.

When this happens, it's said that your body has achieved immunity over a particular threat.

In summary, this is just an overview of how the amazing immune system works to defend your body against outside invaders, including viruses, bacteria, parasites, fungi and much more. There are many other immune system components in this stunning arsenal of defense, including inter-leukins, interferons and much more.

Let's turn now and investigate in-depth these most common of miseries: colds, flu and sinus infections.

Symptoms of Colds, Flu and Sinus Infections

Colds

More than two hundred different viruses can cause the common cold, but the most common ones are rhinoviruses. Colds generally produce symptoms including nasal congestion, sore throat, head congestion, fatigue, weakness, muscle aches and clear mucus drainage. Symptoms usually last seven to ten days.

Colds are commonly confused with allergies or sinus infections. If your symptoms begin quickly and end within one to two weeks, it's most likely you experienced a cold and not an allergy or sinus infection. If the symptoms last more than two weeks, the cold could progress into a sinus infection. Rarely do colds produce fevers or headaches. They will occasionally cause sneezing, a cough and red, watery, itchy eyes. Seasonal allergies, on the other hand, only rarely cause muscle aches and pains, or fatigue. Even less often are they accompanied by a fever or a headache. Seasonal allergies usually produce sneezing with red, watery, itchy eyes, a stuffy nose and occasionally a sore throat.

> *You will keep in perfect peace all who trust in you, whose thoughts are fixed on you!*
> —ISAIAH 26:3

Flu

The symptoms of influenza appear suddenly and often include a fever of 100 degrees to 104 degrees Fahrenheit, and it may reach 106 degrees Fahrenheit. The fever usually is continuous, but it may come and go. In addition, flu sufferers may experience shaking chills; body and muscle aches (often severe), commonly in the back, arms or legs; headache; pain when moving the eyes; fatigue and malaise; loss of appetite; a dry cough; runny noise; and a dry or sore throat.[1]

Epidemics of the flu are very common during the winter months, and flu viruses are extremely contagious. Getting the flu also makes you more susceptible to ear infections, sinusitis and pneumonia.

Flu season is so common that many of us have learned to take these outbreaks in stride, when, in fact, flu is a major national killer. It is linked to about 20,000 deaths in the U.S. each year, and about 130,000 people go to a hospital each year with the flu. Serious respiratory infections, including the flu and pneumonia, are the fifth leading cause of death in individuals sixty-five years of age and older.

Sinusitis

Chronic sinusitis is the most common chronic disease in the U.S., affecting about 40 million people. Studies reveal that the vast majority of individuals with chronic colds lasting longer than two weeks actually have a sinus infection.[2]

If you have suffered from a sinus infection, it was one of two types: acute or chronic sinusitis.

Acute sinusitis is usually triggered by a cold. Symptoms of acute sinusitis include a cold that lasts longer than two weeks, yellow or green nasal drainage, a fever, cough, postnasal drip, facial pressure—especially around the cheeks or eyes or forehead—pain in the upper molars and swelling of the face. Some people experience loss of the sense of smell. There's a good possibility that your sinuses are infected if pain occurs after tapping your cheekbones, the area around the bridge of your nose or your forehead just over the eyebrows.

Chronic sinusitis usually produces fewer symptoms than acute sinusitis. Symptoms include nasal congestion, postnasal drainage, sore throat, cough, low-grade fever, decreased sense of taste and smell and constant cold symptoms such as a constant runny nose. These symptoms usually will interfere with your sleep.

In 1999, a Mayo Clinic study found that an immune system response to fungus, rather than bacterial infection, is the cause of most cases of chronic sinusitis. These researchers studied 210 patients with chronic sinusitis and found forty different kinds of fungus, including candida, in the mucus of 96 percent of the patients.

However, in a control group of healthy volunteers, similar organisms were found as well. Therefore, researchers concluded the immune systems of those with chronic sinusitis reacted dramatically differently than those of healthy individuals.

The unusual immune reaction was determined

to be responsible for the chronic pain, inflammation and swelling of the mucous membranes associated with sinusitis. This is now actually termed "allergic fungal sinusitis." And again, it's an immune system response and not an allergy to the fungus that is the cause of chronic sinus infection.[3]

Divine Health and Colds, Flu and Sinus Infections

Understanding the amazing shield of defense God has provided for your body is a key factor in walking in God's divine health. A healthy, intact immune system can take on even the most deadly assaults of cancer, hepatitis and any other killer that may be lurking in your environment. Colds, flu and sinus infections pose little challenge to a healthy, well-functioning immune system operating at peak efficiency. It may even surprise you to realize that your immune system already is handling many of these invaders with ease.

You see, the immune system is a strong and ready defender for your body, but instead of working with it, often we work against it, sabotaging and undermining its power. God says, "My people are destroyed for lack of knowledge" (Hos. 4:6, KJV). In few places is this so true as with modern living and our immune system.

As you will see throughout the following chapters of this book, by understanding, supporting and supplying the immune system, you can help your body build up your defenses in order to walk in divine health.

A BIBLE CURE PRAYER
FOR YOU

Dear Lord, thank You that I am fearfully and wonderfully made. Your wisdom is beyond all human comprehension, and in Your foreknowledge You designed my body with fantastic resources for divine health. If in ignorance I have sabotaged my own immune system, I ask You to open the eyes of my understanding and make me wise. I repent for my ignorance, and I thank You for teaching me Your ways and plan for walking in divine health. In Jesus' name, amen.

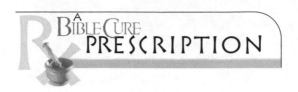

Faith Builder

He was pierced through for our trans-
gressions, He was crushed for our iniq-
uities; the chastening for our well-being
fell upon Him, and by His scourging we
are healed.

—Isaiah 53:5, NAS

Personalize this verse. On a sheet of paper, write out
the verse, and insert your name into it.

Below the personalized verse, write out a personal
prayer to Jesus Christ, thanking Him for purchasing
your healing from colds, flu and sinus infections.

Chapter 2

Preparing the Troops— Nutrition

Nehemiah and his men had to rebuild the walls of Jerusalem while the battle raged. He stationed troops both to battle and to build. The Bible says, "And it came about from that day on, that half of my servants carried on the work while half of them held the spears, the shields, the bows, and the breastplates" (Neh. 4:16, NAS).

Just like Nehemiah, you too may need to address the enemies of your health with a two-pronged approach. To experience God's divine health, you may need to both rebuild and fend off the attack simultaneously.

Nutrition is a key factor in this approach. Your immune system—which comprises the walls of defense for your health—is largely dependent upon you to provide it with the proper nourishment it requires to do its job.

The armed forces would never send troops

into battle with food rations of candy and cookies and little else. A conquering force must be sustained and built up with healthy food. Your immune system is no different. It deserves the very best preparation for the daily battle it must wage against germs, viruses and other invaders.

In addition to being built up and strengthened with the right nutrition, certain foods exist that will actually help your body fight off an attack of the cold, flu or sinus infection—the two-pronged

> *Above all else, guard your heart, for it affects everything you do.*
> —PROVERBS 4:23

approach. So, let's turn now and examine how nutrition can help your body win its battle.

Arming Your Body

In order for your immune system to work at peak efficiency, it needs certain nutrients and foods to fuel all its different areas and functions. Can you imagine sending a soldier to battle and simply giving him a pocketknife and a BB gun? In essence, that's what many of us do when we feed our bodies sugar, highly processed carbohydrates, bad fats, fried foods and foods to which we are allergic or sensitive. Certain foods can actually impair the immune system, sabotaging its effectiveness. Sugar is at the top of the list.

Be smart about sugar

High sugar consumption severely impairs your immune system's ability to function. Yet, in 1999 the U.S. Department of Agriculture reported that the average American consumed approximately 150 pounds of sugar per year. The USDA projects that if consumption trends continue at their current rate, added sugar intake may increase as much as 20 percent by the year 2005.

That's more sugar than many people actually weigh. Not only cakes, pies and cookies are loaded with sugar, but sugar is also a hidden ingredient in many other foods such as ketchup, salad dressings and breads. In fact, many consumers are completely unaware that sugar is a main ingredient in hundreds of processed and packaged foods. It comes disguised under terms such as high-fructose corn syrup, barley malt, rice syrup, maple syrup, concentrated juice, beets, honey and more.

A diet high in sugar makes a person more susceptible to colds, flu and sinus infections. In addition, it provides empty calories—no minerals, no vitamins, no antioxidants and no protein. Yet, your immune system depends upon you to supply

17

it with the adequate, health-building materials it needs to keep you healthy.

For almost a century scientists have known that diabetics were more susceptible than nondiabetics to infections. However, in 1942 researchers discovered that diabetics' white blood cells were unusually sluggish.[1]

Further studies have shown that the more sugar an individual eats, the less efficient his or her white blood cells become. Simple sugars have been shown to lower phagocytosis by 50 percent. (You'll recall that phagocytosis is the immune system's second line of defense against viruses and bacteria.)

So, if your breakfast consists of coffee with a few teaspoons of sugar and a doughnut, and your lunch and dinner consist of one or two sodas with your meal plus a large dessert, realize that you are suppressing your immune system. This can open the door to viral and bacterial infections, especially colds, flu and sinus infections. And the more sugar you consume, the greater will be the negative impact on your immune system.

Excessive sugar in the diet is also a main contributor for candida, which is overgrowth of yeast in the intestinal tract. As we'll see in later chapters, many individuals with chronic sinusitis have

have taken many courses of antibiotics, which have left them with candidiasis that is oftentimes overlooked by their doctors.

Please read my book *The Bible Cure for Candida and Yeast Infections* for more information.

Beat the bad fats rap

Most Americans follow the standard American diet, which consists of eating not only way too much sugar, but also refined flour, too much bread and excessive amounts of bad fats. Bad fats include hydrogenated and partially hydrogenated fats. You can find them in the following:

- Vegetable shortening
- Margarine
- Many deep-fried foods
- Most salad dressings
- Cakes
- Pies
- Cookies
- Most processed foods

Refined, polyunsaturated fats such as safflower oil, corn oil, soybean oil and so forth can impair immunity by interfering with the ability of white blood cells to fight infections. Try to limit these "bad fat" items.

A Healthier Way

You wouldn't choose to build a house with inferior materials if you had superior materials at your disposal, would you? Determine to begin choosing healthier building materials for your immune system. Eat foods that can strengthen and build your body and immune system.

Choose foods that are baked, grilled or broiled instead of fried. Light stir-frying in macadamia nut oil, a little organic butter or extra-virgin olive oil is also acceptable.

Prefer monounsaturated fats, such as extra-virgin olive oil, macadamia nut oil, avocados, almonds, olives and macadamia nuts.

Vegetables, fruits and whole grains

Make it a point to eat at least five servings of fresh vegetables and fruits every day. When selecting fruits and vegetables, it's best to select organically grown varieties when possible. They are free from the pesticides, fertilizers, waxes, fumigants and other toxic materials that contaminate our foods and impair immune function.

Hot Lemonade

Here's a great natural treatment for a sore throat.

4 lemons
Several slices ginger root
Stevia to taste

Juice several lemons, then scrub well and peel. Slice thinly, and add to the juice. Add ginger root. Cover all with plenty of boiling water; cover and steep until cool. Strain off the liquid, and add Stevia and additional water to taste. Drink hot.[2]

Dairy products

If you suffer with recurrent sinus infections or chronic sinusitis, you should avoid all dairy products. The protein in these products tends to increase and thicken mucous secretions.

Are You Allergic to Mold?

Many individuals with chronic sinus infections are allergic to molds. If you are one of them, you will find that certain foods will cause nasal congestion right after you eat them.

A mold allergy will cause nasal congestion

when you eat fermented foods (for example, cheese, sour cream, mushrooms, beer, vinegar, wine or leftover foods), as well as foods made with yeast such as most bakery products.

The Wonder of Water

It's vitally important to drink enough filtered water on a daily basis when you're battling colds, flu and sinus infections. Water will keep your respiratory tract well hydrated. It also helps to liquefy any thick mucus that may be present in those with sinus infections.

I recommend drinking at least two quarts of filtered water. Get accustomed to drinking room-temperature water instead of iced water or cold water. Cold liquids can actually impair normal respiratory function.

Chicken Soup for the Immune System

Chicken soup has been called Jewish penicillin for years. But now researchers are discovering what Jewish mothers knew all along. Chicken soup can help a cold or flu. Hot chicken soup will actually help increase the flow of mucus and help clear out your sinuses.

A 1978 study published in the journal *Chest*

found that drinking hot chicken soup increased the nasal mucus velocity in fifteen healthy subjects from an average of 6.9 to 9.2 mm per minute. Chicken soup actually helps speed up the ciliary movement of the nose and bronchial passages so that they can eliminate microbes.[5]

Besides hot chicken soup, hot herbal teas and vegetable broths, certain foods can also thin the mucus and stimulate the flow of mucus. Hot spicy foods such as cayenne pepper, garlic and horseradish all help to clear nasal congestion and promote drainage. A Japanese horseradish called wasabi also promotes nasal drainage.

✓ A BIBLE CURE HEALTHFACT

Wasabi (wasabe), which is also called Japanese horseradish, comes from the root of an Asian plant. It's used to make a green-colored condiment that has a sharp, pungent, hot flavor. It can be found in specialty and Asian markets in both paste and powder form.[4]

HEALTHFACT HEALTHFACT HEALTHFACT HEALTHFACT HEALTHFACT HEALTHFACT HEALTHFACT

Foods to Avoid for Sinus Infections

Just as certain foods can help relieve the miserable symptoms of colds and sinus infections, other foods can work against you.

Cold drinks, ice cream and Popsicles can result in a buildup of mucus in the sinus cavities. In addition, eggs, chocolate, food additives and excessive alcohol can also trigger a buildup of mucus in many individuals.

Rebuilding and Battling

Setting up a guard nutritionally will involve launching a campaign with two objectives: building the wall, or strengthening your immune system with proper nutrition, and eating foods that directly impact the symptoms of your cold, flu or sinus infection. Just like Nehemiah and his men, you will be holding bricks in one hand and a sword in the other.

Realize that as you are setting up a guard, the Lord will be watching, too. Psalm 121:5 says, "The LORD himself watches over you! The LORD stands beside you as your protective shade." His mighty power is at work in you to strengthen and heal you.

A Bible Cure Prayer
FOR YOU

Dear God, I'm grateful for Your wisdom about my immune system and how to strengthen it with the right kinds of nutrition. Grant me the discipline I need to change old, destructive eating habits. You've been so kind and gracious to heal me of every cold and flu. Help me to build my own body like a wise builder so I can truly walk in Your purpose and plan for my life—Your wonderful divine health. Amen.

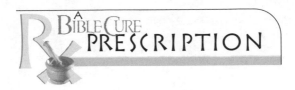

List food items you've been eating that may have contributed to tearing down your immune system.

_____

_____

_____

What items in your list are you willing to give up in order to strengthen your immune system and help it do its job of protecting your body?

_____

_____

_____

How will you work to limit your sugar intake?

_____

_____

_____

Chapter 3

Sending in Supplies—
Supplements

A good general knows one way to conquer an
enemy is to cut off its supply lines. The mightiest force in the world cannot last long without
steady reinforcements of supplies. Supplies and
provision are key factors for gaining victory.

In fact, in ancient times shutting off the supply
lines that fed into the protective walls of a city
was a standard military tactic for defeating an
enemy.

> Some time, later, however, King Ben-
> hadad of Aram mobilized his entire
> army and besieged Samaria. As a result
> there was a great famine in the city. After
> a while even a donkey's head sold for
> two pounds of silver, and a cup of dove's
> dung cost about two ounces of silver.
>
> —2 KINGS 6:24–25

This enemy's military tactic involved weakening Israel's defense by cutting off its supplies. He expected the Israelites to become so weak that they would eventually succumb.

Interestingly, colds, flu and sinus infections attack your body like an invading army, working hard to break down your immune system's walls of protection surrounding your health. During such attacks, massive amounts of nutrients—vitamins, minerals, enzymes, amino acids and more—are required to maintain its strong shield of defense. But when these nutrients are in short supply, your immune system must work even harder to battle invaders without the supplies it needs.

> *For thus saith the Lord GOD, the Holy One of Israel; In returning and rest shall ye be saved; in quietness and in confidence shall be your strength.*
> —ISAIAH 30:15, KJV

But you can send in reinforcements. You can strengthen your body's immune system by taking supplements. Let's turn now and look at a number of supplements that can make all the difference in times of illness and during colds and flu season in general.

Get the Basics

Your body needs to maintain a good, steady supply of basic vitamins and minerals to maintain its fighting edge. Today's modern diet does not always provide all the essentials. In fact, even if your diet is rich with fruits and vegetables, there's a good chance they were grown on depleted soil. Therefore, to maintain the strength and power of your immune system, take a good multivitamin/mineral supplement every day.

A comprehensive multivitamin/mineral

Certain vitamins and minerals are critically important for your immune system to function at peak efficiency, which is vital during cold and flu season. A comprehensive multivitamin is very important to provide the basic vitamins and minerals for your body that it cannot make for itself. You cannot get adequate amounts from the food you eat. Therefore, I recommend a comprehensive multivitamin/mineral supplement such as Divine Health's Elite Multivitamin. It provides essential vitamins and minerals as well as most of the antioxidants your body requires on a daily basis.

Vitamin A

If your body lacks enough vitamin A, you will tend to be very prone to many types of infections, especially colds and flu. Vitamin A works to maintain the structural integrity of the mucous membranes. It's also vitally important in the production of T-cells.

A deficiency of vitamin A will actually cause your thymus gland to shrink, resulting in an impaired immune system. Many physicians are concerned about vitamin A overdosing, since it's associated with liver damage, loss of hair, headaches, vomiting and other symptoms. Yet, vitamin A overdosing is extremely rare, but inadequate consumption of vitamin A is very common.

I recommend approximately 5,000 to 10,000 I.U. of vitamin A every day, which is a safe dosage. However, if you are pregnant, limit your dosage to 5,000 I.U. of vitamin A per day.

Some people believe they don't need vitamin A because they take supplements of beta carotene. They reason that since beta carotene is a precursor to vitamin A, it's all they really need. However, vitamin A, beta carotene and other carotenoids all have independent roles to play in strengthening and protecting immunity. Therefore, all of these nutrients should be taken regularly. Vitamin A is present in most multivitamins.

B-complex

B vitamins are also very important for optimal immune function. Vitamin B_5, or pantothenic acid, is important for maintaining a healthy thymus gland and for antibody production. Folic acid is important for optimal function of T-cells and B-cells, as is vitamin B_6. Vitamin B_{12} is needed by phagocytes to kill bacteria.

A comprehensive multivitamin should have adequate doses of B-complex.

The RDA for B vitamins is rather low, in my opinion. Therefore, I recommend for my patients at least 25 mg of the following B vitamins: vitamin B_1 (thiamine), vitamin B_2 (riboflavin), vitamin B_3 (niacin), vitamin B_5 (pantothenic acid) and vitamin B_6 (pyridoxine). I also recommend at least the following doses of the other B vitamins: folic acid, 800 mcg; vitamin B_{12} and biotin, 100 mcg.

Vitamin C

Vitamin C is also extremely important for the immune system. Vitamin C is both an antiviral and antibacterial agent. Vitamin C strengthens connective tissue and also neutralizes toxic substances that are released from phagocytes.

In 1970 Dr. Linus Pauling released the book *Vitamin C and the Common Cold.*[1] He was one of the most prominent and respected scientists of the twentieth century and had been awarded two Nobel prizes. But he stirred up tremendous controversy in the medical community when he recommended that people take 1,000 to 2,000 mg of vitamin C daily for general well-being. To fight a cold, he recommended upping the dosage to 4,000 to 10,000 mg a day.

Dr. Pauling found that supplementing with 1,000 mg of vitamin C daily reduced the incidence of colds by 45 percent and reduced cold symptoms by 63 percent.[2]

> *My people are destroyed for lack of knowledge.*
> —HOSEA 4:6, KJV

As a preventive dose, I recommend 1,000 mg of vitamin C taken daily, preferably 250 mg three to four times a day or 500 mg twice a day.

If you have a cold or sinus infection, I recommend boosting your dosage to 2,000 mg of vitamin C, preferably in powdered form, every two to three hours. Maintain this dosage for several days, and then gradually taper off until you're back to 1,000 mg a day as a maintenance dose.

Taking over 3,000 mg of vitamin C at one time is likely to produce diarrhea and gas. If you experience such symptoms, decrease your dose to only 500–1,000 mg. In rare instances, high doses of vitamin C can cause kidney stones; therefore, it's critically important to drink at least two quarts of filtered water a day.

Consult with your physician before starting a high-dose vitamin C therapy. Divine Health Buffered Vitamin C contains 700 mg per dose and is an excellent way to strengthen your immune system.

Selenium

Minerals are also vitally important for good immune function. One of the most important minerals for building and maintaining superior immunity is selenium. Selenium deficiency causes a reduction in T-cell activity and antibody production. It can also lower your resistance to developing viral and bacterial infections.

Selenium supplements significantly enhance the body's production of white blood cells—especially T-cells and natural killer cells.

Take approximately 200 mcg of selenium a day.

A comprehensive multivitamin contains selenium.

Zinc

Zinc is another very important mineral for the immune system. In fact, it's the most important mineral to the thymus gland. Zinc is required for cell-mediated immunity, and a deficiency in zinc will cause a decrease in T-cells, natural killer cells and thymic hormone. In test tubes, zinc has been found to prevent cold viruses from reproducing themselves.

A study on zinc throat lozenges found that when subjects who were developing cold symptoms dissolved zinc lozenges in their mouths every two hours, they recovered much faster.[3] Those who took the lozenges recovered in an average of 4.4 days compared with 7.6 days for those who were given a placebo.

Most American diets are low in zinc. Some experts believe our low zinc intake is the reason so many of us have immune problems.

Nevertheless, all zinc is not equal. Zinc gluconate or zinc acetate is preferred to zinc picolinate or zinc citrate. Make sure that your zinc throat lozenges do not contain sugar, citrate or tartrate fillers, since zinc binds to these fillers and becomes less available.

Zinc is also available in a nasal gel called Zicam. Research suggests that the length and severity of a cold may be cut in half when treated with zinc nasal spray within two days of the onset of symptoms.

Whether you elect to use zinc nose spray or zinc throat lozenges, it's important that you begin within twenty-four hours of the first sign of symptoms for the maximum benefit. Zinc is present in a comprehensive multivitamin. I recommend at least 15 mg a day.

Natural Remedies

Let's turn now and look at some natural remedies that can help you beat the symptoms of a cold, flu or sinus infection after you have already become ill.

Echinacea

Historically, Native Americans commonly used echinacea as a medicinal herb. In the 1880s, American physicians started prescribing it but quit in the early part of the twentieth century. In the 1930s, German doctors rediscovered the herb, and it has remained popular overseas since that time.

There are three different species of the plant: *E. angustifolia*, *E. purpurea*, and *E. pallida*. Germany's Commission E, the government agency charged with investigating herbs, recommends treating colds with *E. purpurea*.

Echinacea boosts the immune system's response to colds, flu and other infections. Echinacea is most commonly used in the treatment of the common cold. Start taking it as soon as you notice any cold symptoms.

Take echinacea for three weeks, followed by one week off for best results. Generally speaking, you should take echinacea the same way as you would take an antibiotic.

Don't take echinacea if you are allergic to ragweed. In addition, don't take echinacea if you have an autoimmune disease such as lupus, rheumatoid arthritis, multiple sclerosis or any other autoimmune disease. Do not take echinacea if you are pregnant.

I recommend echinacea purpurea. Take a dosage of 200 mg three times a day of the standardized extract over a two- to three-week period.

Elderberry

Native Americans also used tea made from elderberry flowers to treat respiratory infections. Elderberry extract contains a high percentage of three flavonoids that have been shown to have antiviral properties.

A study published in the *Journal of Alternative and Complementary Medicine* in 1995 examined the flu-fighting capabilities of Sambucol, which is an elderberry extract preparation. The study found that elderberry interfered with the growth of multiple strains of influenza A and B viruses in cell cultures.[4]

During a flu outbreak in an Israeli kibbutz, twenty-seven subjects were given either elderberry or a placebo for three days. The results were amazing: 90 percent of those taking elderberry were completely cured within three days, while most of those who took the placebo needed six days to recover.[5]

> *Or don't you know that your body is the temple of the Holy Spirit, who lives in you and was given to you by God? You do not belong to yourself.*
> —1 CORINTHIANS 6:19

I recommend a standardized extract of elderberry. Take 2–4 tablespoons daily of Black Elderberry Extract, or as directed by your physician. See appendix to order.

Oscillococcinum

Oscillococcinum is the number one over-the-counter flu medication in France, where it has been used for over sixty years. Oscillococcinum

37

is a homeopathic mixture containing a diluted extract of duck liver and heart and comes in granule form. Studies have shown that oscillococcinum may reduce the duration of the illness and severity of the symptoms. A study reported in the April 1998 issue of *British Homeopathic Journal* said 17.4 percent of those taking oscillococcinum were symptom free the day after treatment began compared to only 6 percent of those taking placebos.[6]

This remedy is to be used at the first sign of the flu, preferably within the first eight hours of symptoms, and can be found in most health food stores. Follow the instructions on the package for dosage.

Proteolytic enzymes

Proteolytic enzymes are anti-inflammatory agents that are extremely effective in treating sinusitis. Bromelain is a proteolytic enzyme found in pineapple juice and the stems of the pineapple plants.

In 1993, Germany's Commission E approved bromelain for reducing swelling of the nose and sinuses caused by injuries and operations.

A typical dosage of bromelain is 500 mg three times a day taken between meals on an empty stomach.

Divine Health Proteolytic Enzymes contain two proteolytic enzymes: pancreatin and bromelain. Take three tablets in the morning and three in the evening on an empty stomach. See appendix to order.

Papaya and bromelain enzyme tablets also may help to relieve sinus congestion and eustachian tube blockage. Clear-Ease is an enzyme product that contains bromelain and papaya enzymes. It actually contains one million enzyme units of bromelain and 500,000 units of papaya. It is recommended that you melt this in the mouth three times a day.

Phytosterols

One of the most important supplements in preventing colds, flu and sinus infections is phytosterols. Sterols are plant fats that are similar to the animal fat cholesterol. All plants—including vegetables, fruits, nuts and seeds—contain sterols and sterolins.

These sterols play a very important role in immune activity. Phytosterols can help T-cells multiply. In fact, one study showed T-cell response to this substance increasing from 20 percent to 920 percent after only four weeks on the sterol/sterolin mixture.

Another experiment showed dramatic increases in natural killer cell activity. I've found phytosterols very effective in protecting many individuals against developing colds, flu and sinus infections.

You can obtain phytosterols in an over-the-counter product called Moducare. I recommend one tablet three times a day, one hour before meals, or two in the morning and one in the evening on an empty stomach.

Another powerful phytosterol is Natur-Leaf. Take one tablet twice a day on an empty stomach. See appendix to order.

Olive leaf extract

In Ezekiel God speaks of a tree. "All kinds of fruit trees will grow along both sides of the river. The leaves of these trees will never turn brown and fall, and there will always be fruit on their branches. There will be a new crop every month, without fail! For they are watered by the river flowing from the Temple. The fruit will be for food and the leaves for healing" (Ezek. 47:12).

A bitter substance called *oleuropein* has been isolated from the olive leaf. The active ingredient in oleuropein has been found to possess powerful antibacterial properties as well as to inhibit the growth of viruses. The olive leaf has the ability to interrupt the replication of many different pathogens, including bacteria and viruses. It has been found to be effective in treating the flu, colds and sinus infections.

The dose of this extract typically is 500 mg every six hours taken between meals. For acute infections, some physicians recommend two tablets every six hours.

Colloidal silver

You have probably heard the expression, "He was born with a silver spoon in his mouth." It comes from the awful days of the plagues in Europe when no antibiotics or other medicines existed to stop the murderous rampage of disease that wiped out entire towns. Wealthier babies were given silver spoons to suck on throughout the day. The silver in the spoons provided an antibiotic effect, giving these infants a better chance at survival.

Today, silver is still valued for its medicinal powers. Colloidal silver is a clear liquid composed of 99.9 percent pure silver particles, which are about 0.001 to 0.01 microns in diameter and are suspended in pure water.

Colloidal silver has been shown to be effective against more than 650 different pathogens. I especially recommend colloidal silver for sinus infections. I have found it best to use it with a nose dropper three to four times a day in each nostril.

Personally, I consider Sovereign Silver to be a superior colloidal silver product. It can be found in many health food stores. I do not recommend that you ingest colloidal silver; only use it as a nasal solution.

Xlear

Xlear contains xylitol, which is a naturally occurring sugar alcohol found in many fruits and vegetables that tastes and looks just like sugar. Xylitol has actually been used in foods since the 1960s and has been shown to reduce cavities by up to 80 percent.

This substance causes bacteria to lose their grip on the body's membranes, rendering them unable to grow. Once its hold is broken, xylitol then helps to flush the harmful bacteria away.

> *For the angel of the LORD guards all who fear him, and he rescues them.*
> —PSALM 34:7

Antibiotics tend to kill both good and bad bacteria, and they give rise to resistant bacteria growth. Xlear contains xylitol and is an excellent treatment for sinus infections. It is also very safe to use in children. See appendix to order.

Saventaro

Saventaro is a form of cat's claw, an herb used by the people in the Andes, especially in Peru, to treat ailments including infections, arthritis, dysentery and inflammation. Cat's claw contains alkaloids that stimulate the immune system. Its active ingredient is a group of compounds called "pentacyclic oxindole alkaloids," also known as POAs.

Saventaro is the first and only form of cat's claw that comes from the root where the POAs are far more concentrated. This makes this product much more potent than regular cat's claw.

For colds, flu and sinus infections, take two capsules three times a day for seven to ten days. See appendix to order.

Medications and Vaccines for the Flu

In addition to vitamins, supplements and natural remedies, your cold, flu or sinus infection may be severe enough to use a prescription medication. Two new prescription medications are extremely effective in treating the flu by attacking the flu virus and preventing it from spreading inside the body. In other words, they don't just treat flu symptoms, but they actually attack the virus if taken early enough in the course of the infection.

These are Tamiflu and Relenza.

I personally prefer Tamiflu for my patients. It has antiviral activity against influenza A and B. Tamiflu can be taken by patients one year of age and older. However, treatment should begin within two days of the onset of symptoms. If you have symptoms of the flu and can see your doctor within the first two days of symptoms, ask him about prescribing Tamiflu for you or your children.

FluMist

FluMist is an intranasal flu vaccine that contains live (attenuated) influenza viruses. There is, however, a possibility that the weakened viruses can cause the flu, especially in individuals with a weakened immune system. FluMist is approved for use only in healthy individuals between the ages of five and forty-nine. Also, people who have received FluMist should avoid close contact with immunocompromised people for at least twenty-one days. They include people with cancer, HIV and AIDS; individuals on steroid medications; many with autoimmune disease; organ transplant recipients and so on. If you live with an immunocompromised patient and receive FluMist, you are putting them at risk of contracting the flu. I feel it is much safer to get the flu vaccine, which contains killed viruses, as compared to FluMist, which contains live but weakened viruses.

Flu vaccine

The flu vaccine is an injection that contains killed viruses; therefore, you cannot get the flu from the vaccine. It actually contains three different strains of the flu virus. The strains that are chosen each year are the ones that scientists believe are most likely to be present in the U.S. that year. If their choice is correct, the vaccine is 70–90 percent effective in preventing the flu in healthy patients under sixty-five years of age. The flu vaccine is recommended for adults and children over six months of age.

The flu vaccine contains the preservative thimerosal, which contains about 50 percent mercury by weight. There are thimerosal-free vaccines that your physician can order. Especially for young children, I would recommend the thimerosal-free vaccine. I also recommend the thimerosal-free flu vaccine for adults; however, adults are not nearly as susceptible to the harmful effects of thimerosal as young children are. Some researchers believe thimerosal may be linked to autism in children.[7]

It is recommended that you get the flu vaccine each year if:

- You are a healthcare worker
- You have diabetes, heart disease or other long-term health problems
- You have a suppressed immune system
- You have problems with your kidneys
- You have a lung problem such as asthma or emphysema
- You are over fifty, and especially if you are over sixty-five[8]

Honoring Your Body

The Bible says that your body is a temple of the Holy Spirit. "Or don't you know that your body is the temple of the Holy Spirit, who lives in you and was given to you by God? You do not belong to yourself" (1 Cor. 6:19).

As such, honoring your body and caring for it shows your respect and honor for the One who created it. Your immune system is a strong and ready defender for your body, the magnificent work of a divine Creative Genius.

Make it your determination to supply your body with the vitamins, minerals, enzymes, amino acids and all the other building materials it needs to maintain a strong and healthy guard for your health.

Most of all, never stop looking to Jesus Christ as the true source of all healing power.

A BIBLE CURE PRAYER
FOR YOU

Dear Jesus Christ, thank You for being the Healer of my body. Give me the wisdom I need to arm my immune system with all of the materials it needs to work at maximum efficiency. Teach me to maintain the supply lines of health to my body. More than anything, Jesus, teach me to always look to You as my Healer and my Friend. In Jesus' name, amen.

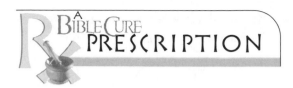
A BIBLE CURE PRESCRIPTION

Circle the supplements you are planning to take to strengthen your immune system after reading this chapter.

Multivitamin/mineral	Zinc
Vitamin C	Selenium
Vitamin A	B-complex

Circle the supplement or herb you may try after reading about them in this chapter.

Echinacea	Elderberry
Phytosterols	Saventaro
Xlear	Colloidal silver
Olive leaf extract	Oscillococcinum

Write a commitment to God expressing what you intend to do to help keep the walls of protection for your health strong and vigorous.

_____

_____

_____

Chapter 4

Ready for Battle—Lifestyle Factors

We wouldn't send our soldiers to war and have them fight battles twenty-four hours a day, seven days a week. We would give them rest—at least some rest every night, and then send in fresh troops every so often. Rest is a principle of God's wisdom. The Bible says, "In returning and rest shall ye be saved; in quietness and in confidence shall be your strength" (Isa. 30:15, KJV).

Your immune system is at war every day, battling germs, viruses and diseases of which you're probably completely unaware. To support and assist your immune system, you must learn to give it rest so that it can be restored and repaired.

Rest is merely one lifestyle factor you must consider in order to prepare and maintain your immune system so it's ready for battle. There are many others that we will examine in this chapter on lifestyle factors.

Are You Guilty?

Getting enough sleep is absolutely critical for maintaining a strong immune system. Lack of sleep causes a decline of natural killer cells. Deep sleep actually helps to strengthen the immune system and repair any tissue damage.

In fact, colds, flu and sinus infections tend to make us feel sleepy for a good reason. When the immune system is battling these germs and viruses, it produces chemicals called *cytokines*, which cause the body to feel tired and sleepy. Our body works to conserve energy so that the immune system can mount up an attack against the infection.

> *He will not let you stumble and fall; the one who watches over you will not sleep.*
> —PSALM 121:3

Unfortunately, too many of us work forty-plus hours a week; when we catch a cold, come down with the flu or develop a sinus infection, we keep pushing ourselves. Does that sound like you?

When you keep pushing yourself when your body is signaling you to sleep, you are undermining your immune system and sabotaging your health. God created principles of health within your body that you need to obey. Cheating your body again and again ultimately can cause disastrous consequences.

When you're ill, make sure that you take time to rest so that your body can heal.

Exercise and Your Immune System

Sleep is vital, both to protect and maintain a powerful immune system. But did you realize that exercise is also very important?

Aerobic exercise is an excellent way to stimulate the immune system and help to prevent infections. Regular exercise will help keep your immune system strong and healthy.

Nevertheless, if you have a cold, flu or sinus infection, you will need to limit your exercise until you recover. I recommend you continue with very light exercise when you are sick, such as some walking. But if you have the flu, stop exercises altogether until you recover.

Regular aerobic exercise helps to decrease stress hormones and drain the sinuses by supplying more blood flow to the nasal area. It also increases mucous secretions so that stagnant mucus can be expelled from the sinus cavities.

Here's another way aerobic exercise works to keep you well. It raises your body's temperature, and heat actually activates the immune system. When you walk briskly or bike for about thirty minutes, your heightened temperature helps to stimulate the immune system. Exercise also oxygenates and strengthens tissues, making them more able to resist infection.

Toxins in the body are eliminated through exercise. Your lymphatic system is vitally important in this elimination process, and it also helps to maintain your body's immune defenses. This system includes the lymph nodes, which are filters placed strategically throughout your body. Each one of us has about six hundred of them that systematically cleanse the body from disease.

> *The LORD himself watches over you! The LORD stands beside you as your protective shade.*
> —PSALM 121:5

Lymph nodes contain white blood cells that scan the lymphatic fluid for bacteria, viruses, organic debris and other microbes. These white blood cells contain much of the immune system's battalion of defense, which we have already discussed. Macrophages, T-cells, B-cells and lymphocytes attack enemy viruses, fungi and bacteria.

When the lymphatic system becomes sluggish or

blocked, the work of white blood cells slows down. Their work of killing invading viruses, bacteria and other microbes is impeded. As a result, infection and disease can more readily take root in the body.

Nevertheless, regular aerobic exercise can supercharge this system, increasing its lymphatic flow threefold. That means three times as much cellular waste and foreign microbes are removed. This, in turn, greatly assists the immune system in its work.

If you do not have a regular aerobic routine, why not make a commitment to start one today? Let's turn now and look at some practical ways you can guard your body against colds, flu and sinus infections.

Lessons From SARS

In November 2002, the first case of a new strain of viral infection was first reported in China. SARS, or "Severe Acute Respiratory Syndrome," is a new viral infection that usually leads to pneumonia. A few isolated cases of SARS were reported in the Toronto area. However, in March 2003, it progressed to a large outbreak in Toronto. This outbreak occurred after a single traveler returned from Hong Kong in late February.

SARS spread from China to more than two dozen countries in North America, South America, Europe and Asia. During the SARS outbreak from February to July 2003, a total of 8,437 people worldwide became ill, and 813 individuals died, according to the World Heath Organization.[1]

In the United States it was reported that 182 people contracted SARS, all of whom improved. Fortunately, the SARS global outbreak of 2003 was contained.[2] However, the World Heath Organization has issued a warning that the illness could reemerge. The symptoms of SARS are very similar to the flu in that people will have a high fever, headache, body aches and overall discomfort, and usually a dry cough. However, most patients develop pneumonia.

This deadly viral infection is much worse than the flu and does not respond to antibiotics. That's why it's critically important to know how this terrible infection is transmitted.

SARS is spread mainly by close person-to-person contact. The virus is passed through respiratory droplets, produced when a person sneezes or coughs. If these droplets land on any of the mucous membranes of your mouth, eyes or nose, or if you touch a surface contaminated with these droplets and then touch your eyes, mouth or nose, you can become infected.

What Can You Do?

Hand washing is the most important method of protecting yourself against SARS as well as other viral and bacterial infections. Along with frequent hand washing, it is also critically important to strengthen your immune system, as we have seen.

The Importance of Hand Washing

Colds, flu and sinus infections are spread when you shake hands with someone or touch an infected surface or object and then touch your nose, eyes or mouth. But hand washing breaks this chain of infection.

An article at CBSNews.com reports that over 100,000 deaths were linked to hospital infections in 2000. "Many of the deaths were caused by unsanitary facilities, germ-laden instruments and *unwashed hands*" (emphasis added).[3] The article mentioned an incident where a doctor dropped a surgical glove on a dirty floor, then picked it up and put it on his hand. He then changed the dressing on an open wound on a burn patient.[4]

Public restrooms are another haven for micro-organisms. After using a public restroom, it's very important to wash your hands with hot water and soap. Use paper towels instead of automatic hand dryers if available. Do not touch the faucet when you turn it off, but use your paper towel to turn it off instead. Then use the same paper towel to open the door or to turn the doorknob. Remember that all the people who didn't wash their hands on the way out have already handled that doorknob.

Do you still use public payphones at the airport or bus station? If so, consider that you are holding the germs of everyone who has used that phone right up against your mouth. It's best to handle public phones with a tissue or handkerchief, and keep the mouthpiece far from your mouth. Remember that they are breeding grounds for germs.

An Innocent Handshake?

It is an American custom to greet someone with a firm handshake. If we would bow as the Orientals do instead of shaking hands, it's very possible that we wouldn't pass around nearly as many infectious diseases. During cold season it may be a good idea to carry antiseptic wipes with you and wipe your hands after shaking hands with individuals or make it a habit to wash them repeatedly throughout the day.

Cold viruses can typically survive for three hours on surfaces, on objects and especially on hands. You see, viruses and bacteria are on our skin, and when we touch our mucous membranes, they easily gain entrance into our bodies.

The simplest measure to prevent colds, flu and sinus infections is to wash your hands frequently. The more often you wash your hands, the fewer colds, flu and sinus infections you get.

In addition to becoming vigilant—although not obsessive—about guarding your exposure to germs and viruses, you also will need to respond with godly wisdom when you contract colds, flu and sinus infections. One of the surest ways to undermine the power of your immune system is to offer the incorrect remedy when treating an illness.

Antibiotics—When NOT to Take Them!

When people have a sinus infection, cold or flu, they generally start taking antibiotics. Either they open an unfinished prescription from their medicine cabinet, or they go to their physician, who is quick to prescribe them. Most people believe that antibiotics will cure their disease.

Many doctors prescribe antibiotics for sore throats, even though the vast majority of sore throats are viral. Only a small percentage is strep throat. Colds and flu stem from viruses, and antibiotics cannot kill them and should not be used. A sinus infection is a bacterial infection, but even then antibiotics can be over-prescribed and overused.

Antibiotics are a double-edged sword. When used too frequently, bacteria can eventually become immune to the antibiotic. This is called "antibiotic resistance." Today, we're seeing more and more antibiotic-resistant strains of bacteria. And physicians are actually helping to breed these super-germs by over-prescribing antibiotics. Overuse of antibiotics weakens the immune system and makes you more vulnerable to repeated illness by breeding a hybrid strain of super-bacteria in your body.

> *He rebuked the wind and said to the water, "Quiet down!" Suddenly the wind stopped, and there was a great calm.*
> —MARK 4:39

According to studies, a single bacterium can regenerate and form over a million bacteria in a span of only six hours. So as you can see, antibiotics are not the answer for this epidemic of chronic sinusitis. The more antibiotics you use, the faster antibiotic-resistant bacteria grow.

Approximately 40 to 50 percent of all antibiotic use in the U.S. today is actually misuse according to some experts.[5] Overuse of antibiotics is one of the main reasons why we're seeing an epidemic of chronic sinusitis. In a 1999 study reported in the Mayo Clinic Proceedings, allergic fungal sinusitis was reported as the cause of chronic sinusitis in the vast majority of cases.[6] Antibiotics are effective against bacterial infections, but not against fungal infections. In fact, many times antibiotics worsen fungal infections by destroying most of the good bacteria in the GI tract and cause one to develop chronic candidiasis.

Therefore, reject the mind-set that reaches for an antibiotic every time you feel pain or pressure over your sinuses. In fact, I've found that most sinus infections can be overcome without antibiotics by simply using natural means.

Triggers of Sinus Infections

The most common triggers to sinus infections are allergies (especially in children) and colds.

When you get a cold, your nasal mucous membrane becomes inflamed, swollen and irritated. The entire lining of the nose and sinuses is covered with a thin coat of mucus. That mucus is sticky and collects airborne particles. It contains enzymes that destroy many bacteria.

The cilia are tiny hairs that line the sinuses and respiratory passages, which sweep away the debris that has been collected by the mucus out of the respiratory passages and sinuses. Anything that impairs the function of the cilia or the mucus can trigger a sinus infection. In addition, factors that cause the mucous glands to secrete more mucus or that create swollen tissues that block drainage can trigger a sinus infection, too.

> *The LORD gives his people strength. The LORD blesses them with peace.*
> —PSALM 29:11

A cold virus shuts down the cilia, causing mucus in the nose to stagnate. Dry air from heaters and furnaces during cold winter months makes it worse. Cold air and frigid temperatures further irritate and injure the cilia, which is what triggers a runny nose. So you can see, many different factors work against the movement of the cilia and sets you up for a sinus infection.

When mucous membranes become inflamed, swollen and irritated, the mucous glands secrete even more mucus. Mucus normally drains easily through sinus openings, but if the membranes become swollen, irritated and inflamed, the mucus can't drain out. It becomes stagnant and easily infected.

If the mucus doesn't drain efficiently, the person will experience quite a bit of facial pressure, swelling and pain over the sinus cavities.

Structural problems can also contribute to sinus infections. You may have a deviated nasal septum that hinders proper drainage. Nasal polyps inside the nasal cavity are growths that look similar to grapes and set up sinus infections by obstructing nasal drainage.

It's not clear why nasal polyps develop. Some may be caused by allergies, while others may be triggered by aspirin, chemicals or even infections. But polyps commonly return. If you suffer from nasal polyps, your doctor may prescribe one of the new low-dose steroid nasal sprays, which are effective in keeping polyps from returning.

Many factors can both cause and trigger sinus infections. By recognizing the irritating factors, you can then take measures to protect your cilia and mucous membranes from an assault.

Know Your Nose

Besides the sense of smell, the nose and sinuses have a very important function. They filter, humidify and regulate the temperature of the air you breathe in. If the mucous membrane becomes irritated or infected, a cold or a sinus infection may occur. Therefore, making sure your sinuses get adequate moisture is extremely important to soothe and relieve irritated mucous membranes, to restore normal ciliary function and to relieve nasal and head congestion, headaches and sore throats.

Using a saline or saltwater nasal spray can provide moisture. You can purchase one over the counter, or you can make your own saline wash.

A BIBLE CURE HEALTH TIP

Make Your Own Saline Wash

You will need:
  2 cups or 1 pint warm water
  1 tsp. salt (sea salt or kosher salt is preferred)
  $1/2$ tsp. baking soda

Mix ingredients together. Rinse out nasal cavities three to four times per day when suffering from an acute sinus infection. Twice per day for chronic sinusitis.

Try using a Neti Pot for irrigation. Use a full cup of saline solution per each irrigation. A Neti Pot is a ceramic container that you can purchase at many health food stores that looks similar to a genie's magic lamp. Just fill it up with the saline solution, lean over the sink, and tilt your head to one side as you pour the solution directly into one nostril with the Neti Pot. The solution will run out the other nostril and run down the back of your throat.

More Natural Treatments for Sinus Infections

Grossan Pulsatile Nasal Irrigator

Another method of saline irrigation uses the Grossan Pulsatile Nasal Irrigator. This device attaches to a Waterpik appliance. Dr. Murray Grossan is an ENT specialist who specializes in treating scuba divers' ear, nose and throat problems. He developed the Pulsatile Nasal Irrigator as a drug-free approach for treating sinusitis and blocked eustachian tubes. For more information on the Grossan Pulsatile Nasal Irrigator, please visit his Web site at www.ent-consult.com.

Steam baths

Steam baths are an excellent way to provide moisture to your mucous membranes and nasal cavities. Or simply take a very hot, steamy shower and inhale the steam. It's very important to breathe the steam in through your nose to get the beneficial effects.

You may also purchase a steam inhaler that uses a plastic mask that covers your nose and mouth.

Eucalyptus oil

Eucalyptus oil is another very good method to help clear your sinus congestion. Simply use it as directed. You can find it at many health food stores.

Simmering saline water

If you do not have access to steam, a steam bath or a steam inhaler, you may simply try keeping a pot of saline water simmering on the stove. As you cook or work around the house, stop and lean over the pot and inhale the steam for several minutes at a time. This is a very inexpensive way of providing moisture to your nasal passages.

Shower massage

A very effective, inexpensive way to soothe sinus congestion and pressure is by simply replacing your showerhead with a shower massage. While taking a shower, set the shower massage on a pulsating setting and allow very warm water to pulsate over your sinus cavities. This provides dramatic relief for many of my sinus sufferers.

Remember, Moisture Is Key

For sinus infections, colds and flu, getting enough moisture into your body and sinuses is a key factor in aiding your body to beat the battle. As mentioned earlier, don't forget to drink lots of water to keep your body well hydrated. Don't let your home get dry during winter months. Use a humidifier, or keep a teapot simmering throughout the day to keep moisture in the air. For sinus pain, place a moist, hot cloth over your face.

Guarding the Treasure of Your Good Health

Too many people do not value the treasure of good health until they lose it. As a medical doctor, I see a side of life that most individuals don't get to see. I hear the regret and sense of loss of those who no longer enjoy vital health. Sadly, so much of the suffering I see is unnecessary. The old proverb is really true that says an ounce of prevention is worth a pound of cure. Far too many Americans wake up and treasure the gift of good health only after it is gone. Don't be among them.

The Bible says, "Guard, through the Holy Spirit who dwells in us, the treasure which has been entrusted to you" (2 Tim. 1:14, NAS). The good health God has given you is a gift, and He has made you the steward of that gift. Learn to see your health as a treasure from above that you must guard with godly wisdom every day.

A BIBLE CURE PRAYER
FOR YOU

Dear Lord, forgive me for not being the steward of my good health that I should be. Help me to see my health as a treasure to be highly valued and carefully maintained. As with any gift, I acknowledge that I must prove myself worthy of it. Grant me Your wisdom as I endeavor to guard my immune system, to give my body the rest it requires, to eat right, to drink water and to address symptoms of colds, flu and sinus infection early. Help me never to undermine or sabotage my own body's immune system through foolish or unnecessary treatment. In Jesus' name, amen.

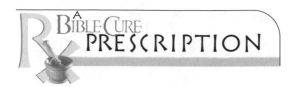

A BIBLE CURE PRESCRIPTION

Describe ways that you have sabotaged or undermined your own immune system's power and efficiency.

———————————————————

———————————————————

———————————————————

How have you failed to be a good steward of your gift of good health?

———————————————————

———————————————————

———————————————————

How much rest does your body require?

———————————————————

How can you give it more rest during illness?

———————————————————

———————————————————

———————————————————

Chapter 5

Guarding Your Heart

Throughout this book, we have discussed a great deal about guarding—guarding your immune system, guarding your health and guarding your activities and lifestyle choices so that you can enjoy the wellspring of vital health God has intended for you. But walking in God's best—His divine health—involves more than the body. He intends for you to be blessed body, mind and spirit. And just as guarding is a powerful principle of physical health, so it is also in the spiritual realm. The Bible says, "Above all else, guard your heart, for it affects everything you do" (Prov. 4:23).

You may be wondering, *How does what goes on in my heart affect whether or not I get a cold, flu or sinus infection?* Well, believe it or not, the impact is greater than you might imagine.

Just as certain foods can impair the immune system, excessive stress can have the same result. Stress also involves your perceptions of events in your life more than the actual events themselves.

Chronic Stress and Immunity

Downsizing in industry is causing more and more individuals to be asked to do more and more work with less time and fewer resources. Benefits are pared down, and employees often get less vacation time. Our electronic age keeps us tied to work through cell phones, beepers, computers and fax machines.

Chronic stress can weaken the immune system. Excessive stress actually causes excessive amounts of cortisol to be produced in your body, which causes the thymus gland to shrink. You'll recall that the thymus gland is critically important for cell-mediated immunity and produces the critically important T-cells. Stress reduces the number of T-cells your immune system has to fight disease. It also decreases the numbers and the activity of natural killer cells.

> *For thus saith the LORD, Behold, I will extend peace to her like a river.*
> —ISAIAH 66:12, KJV

Too much cortisol in your bloodstream can impact the work of the lymph glands. The result of excessive stress chemicals in the body is that the immune system no longer is able to keep infections at bay.

Stress opens the door for infections to enter into the body. I tell my patients that living in stress is similar to leaving your front door open at night. Any snake, possum, skunk or rat can crawl in through your front door and set up a nest in your house.

A similar thing happens with your immune system. When you are under chronic stress, your immune system is weakened, and any bacteria or virus can gain entrance into your body and set up residence in your body—especially in your sinuses.

Perception, Stress and Heart Matters

The problem of stress lies not with circumstances—not really. It's how we perceive and react to those circumstances that stresses us out. That's why one man can sit in his car in heavy traffic and whistle a tune while another one blows his stack. Stressful circumstances represent about 10 percent of a problem. Your reaction to those circumstances comprises the remaining 90 percent.

The Bible says, "You will keep in perfect peace all who trust in you, whose thoughts are fixed on you!" (Isa. 26:3). Perfect peace in stressful circumstances is possible, but it takes work. It requires continually checking your attitude against the Word of God. And it requires faith.

Your perception and reaction to stressful circumstances will determine how your immune system responds. If you respond to trying and difficult circumstances with faith, peace and joy, your immune system will respond with strength. But if you react by feeling depression, anxiety, grief,

> *Those who love your law have great peace and do not stumble.*
> —PSALM 119:165

fear and a loss of control, your immune system will become physically depressed.

However, on the other hand, joy and laughter actually stimulate the immune system. Loma Linda University Medical Center's Dr. Lee Berk reports that laughter helps the immune system in very specific ways:

- It increases IgA, which helps protect against respiratory infections.
- It increases gamma interferons, the immune system's front-line defense against viruses.

- It increases B-cells, which produce antibodies directly against harmful bacteria.
- It increases helper T-cells, which help to organize the immune system's response.
- It increases the number and activity of natural killer cells, which attack tumor cells and viruses.[1]

This is the reason I prescribe ten belly laughs a day for my patients; it stimulates the immune system better than most medicines and supplements—and it is without side effects. Nehemiah 8:10 says, "The joy of the LORD is your strength!" How true this is for our immune system.

Therefore, to strengthen your immune system, strengthen your heart in God's peace, joy and faith. Build up your spirit by reading His powerful Word every day. Stay close to His presence by praying often. For more information on this topic, please refer to my books *The Bible Cure for Stress* and *Deadly Emotions*.

Choose Faith

Every one of us will experience difficulties in this life, but not all of us will let them overwhelm our emotions and destroy our good health. When difficulties come, choose faith.

Faith is not an eerie force or mystical dove. Faith is a choice, and you have all the faith you need right this second to defeat any foe. The Bible says that faith as small as a mustard seed can move mountains. Why? Because faith is a choice.

So, when circumstances seem to be working to get you down, make up your mind to choose faith. Believe in a God who loves you, suffered for you so that you could be healed and gave His own life on a cross so that you could be victorious in every circumstance.

In addition, believe the best. If you hear yourself announce that you get a cold every winter, stop believing for the worst to happen. Expect God's best every day—expect to walk in the blessings of divine health, and you will.

A BIBLE CURE PRAYER
FOR YOU

Dear Lord Jesus, thank You for suffering so that I might be healed. Thank You for dying that I might live. Thank You for enduring the cross so that I might walk in the power of Your victory every day of my life. Today, I choose faith. I make up my mind to believe that You have provided my life with all I need to walk and live in health, safety, peace and joy. I promise to work with Your plan for my life—never against it. Most of all, I praise You with all my heart for being such a wonderful Creator, Father and Friend who loves me with a strength and power I can't even imagine. In Jesus' name, amen.

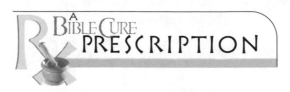

On a sheet of paper, write out a contract with God
promising to live in divine health to the best of your
ability (with His help), to choose a healthy lifestyle
that honors Him and to stop sabotaging or undermining your own health. When you are finished, sign
it and date it.

After writing out the contract, write a prayer
asking God to help you keep your commitment to
divine health.

Conclusion

If you have been having recurrent colds, flu or sinus infections, now you have the information you need to overcome each of these diseases. Realize that an ounce of prevention is worth a pound of cure, and simple, frequent hand washing is absolutely the most important thing that you can do to prevent these infections. Be an example of good hygiene by washing your hands before every meal, and teach your children to do the same.

Begin to strengthen your immune system by changing your diet and dramatically decreasing your consumption of sugar as well as most dairy products if you are sensitive to them. Cultivate good health habits by setting aside time to exercise on a regular basis. Also, make it a priority to get seven to eight hours of sleep each night.

And finally, begin to both decrease your stress and your reactions to stress. Remember that stress is only 10 percent of the problem, but how you react to the stress is the other 90 percent.

Learn to react to stress the way Jesus reacted.

A storm came up and started to fill the boat where the disciples were with water. The disciples ran to Jesus and found Him in deep sleep. When they awakened Him, He rebuked the winds and the rain, and there was a calm. Jesus was always at peace, even in the midst of accusations by the Jewish leaders and the Romans.

By reading God's Word and meditating on it throughout the day, you can renew your mind.

Most importantly, always choose faith. Faith is a power greater than your immune system, greater than any army. For it's by faith that you reach up and touch the Master's hand.

—DON COLBERT, M.D.

Appendix

Saventaro
Call Integrative Therapeutics at 1-800-931-1709 (fax 503-582-0386) to order. Use PCP # 5266.

Xclear
Visit their Web site at www.xclear.com or call 1-877-599-5327.

Natur-Leaf
For more information or to purchase, call Lifeline Inc. at 1-888-532-7845 or 1-505-266-7374. Or e-mail info@naturleaf.com.

Extract of Elderberry
Call Cardiovascular Research at 1-800-888-4585.

Divine Health Vitamin C
Visit our Web site at www.drcolbert.com.

Divine Health Multivitamins
Visit our Web site at www.drcolbert.com.

Divine Health Proteolytic Enzyme
Visit our Web site at www.drcolbert.com.

A Personal Note From
Don and Mary Colbert

God's Word is full of promises that confirm His love for you and His desire to give you His abundant life. His desire includes more than physical health for you; He wants to make you whole in your mind and spirit as well through a personal relationship with His Son, Jesus Christ.

If you haven't met our best friend, Jesus, we would like to take this opportunity to introduce Him to you. It is very simple. Just bow your head and sincerely pray this prayer from your heart:

> *Lord Jesus, I want to know You as my Savior and Lord. I believe You are the Son of God and that You died for my sins. I ask You to forgive me for my sins and change my heart so that I can be Your child and live with You eternally. Thank You for Your peace. Help me to walk with You so that I can begin to know You as my best friend and my Lord. Amen.*

If you have prayed this prayer, we rejoice with you in your decision and your new relationship with Jesus. Please contact us at pray4me@strang.com so that we can send you some materials that will help you become established in your relationship with the Lord. You have just made the most important decision of your life. We look forward to hearing from you.

Notes

PREFACE

1. Robert Ivker, *Sinus Survival* (New York: Jeremy P. Tarcher/Putnam, 2000.)

CHAPTER 1

1. WebMD, "Health Guide A–Z: Influenza," http://my.webmd.com/content/healthwise/75/18578 (accessed December 16, 2003).
2. Ivker, *Sinus Survival.*
3. J. V. Ponike, et al., "The Diagnosis and Incidence of Allergic Fungal Sinusitis," Mayo Clinic proceedings 74 (1999). 877-884.

CHAPTER 2

1. R. Richardson, "Measurement of Phagocytic Activity in Diabetes Mellitus," American Journal of Medical Science (1942): 204–229.
2. Charlotte E. Grayson, M.D., "Can Chicken Soup or Tea Clear My Cold Symptoms?" WebMD, http://my.webmd.com/content/pages/5/4068_105.htm (accessed December 16, 2003).
3. K. Saketkhoo, et al., "Effects of Drinking Hot Water, Cold Water, and Chicken Soup on Nasal Mucus Velocity and Nasal Airflow Resistance," *Chest* 74 (October 1978): 408–410; http://www.ncbi.nlm.nih.gov/entrez/query.fcgi?cmd=Retrieve&db=PubMed&list_uids=359266&

dopt=Abstract (accessed December 16, 2003).

4. Barron's Educational Services, Inc., copyright © 1995, based on Sharon Tyler Herbst, *The Food Lover's Companion*, 2nd edition, s.v. "wasabi," http://eat.epicurious.com/dictionary/food/index.ssf?DEF_ID=4441 (accessed December 16, 2003).

CHAPTER 3

1. Linus Pauling, *Vitamin C and the Common Cold* (San Francisco: W. H. Freeman, 1970).
2. Linus Pauling, "The Significance of the Evidence of Ascorbic Acid and the Common Cold," *Proceedings of the National Academy of Sciences of the USA* 68 (November 1971): 2678-2681.
3. Sherif B. Mossad, et al., "Zinc Gluconate Lozenges for Treating the Common Cold," *Annals of Internal Medicine* 125 (July 15, 1996): 81–88; http://www.annals.org/cgi/content/abstract/125/2/81 (accessed December 16, 2003).
4. Lynda Liu, "Fighting the Flu With Alternative Remedies," January 7, 2000, http://www.cnn.com/2000/HEALTH/01/07/berrying.flu.wmd/index.html (accessed December 16, 2003).
5. Ibid.

6. Ibid.
7. Mark Geier, M.D., Ph.D., and David Geier, "Thimerosal in Childhood Vaccines, Neurodevelopment Disorders and Heart Disease in the United States," *Journal of American Physicians and Surgeons* 8 (Spring 2003): http://www.jpands.org/vol8no1/geier.pdf (accessed December 30, 2003). Also, Kelly Patricia O'Meara, "Vaccines Fueling Autism Epidemic?", *WorldNetDaily*, http://www.worldnetdaily.com/news/article.asp?ARTICLE_ID=32988 (accessed December 30, 2003).
8. Influenza Vaccine, FamilyDoctor.org, http://familydoctor.org/x2084.xml (accessed December 30, 2003).

CHAPTER 4

1. Fact Sheet: Basic Information About SARS, Centers for Disease Control, http://www.cdc.org/ncidod/sars/factsheet.htm (accessed September 8, 2003).
2. Ibid.
3. Hospital Infection Deaths in Focus, CBSNews.com, July 21, 2002, http://www.cbsnews.com/stories/2002/07/20/health/main515755.shtml (accessed December 30, 2003).
4. Ibid.
5. The Immune System—Our Guardian of Health,

http://www.holisticwebs.com/cancer/generic
-report.pdf (accessed December 30, 2003).

6. Ponike, et al., "The Diagnosis and Incidence of Allergic Fungal Sinusitis."

CHAPTER 5

1. L. Berk, "Eustress of Mirthful Laughter Modifies Natural Killer Cell Activity," *Clinical Research* 37 (1989): 115.

Don Colbert, M.D., was born in Tupelo, Mississippi. He attended Oral Roberts University School of Medicine in Tulsa, Oklahoma, where he received a bachelor of science degree in biology in addition to his degree in medicine. Dr. Colbert completed his internship and residency with Florida Hospital in Orlando, Florida. He is board certified in family practice and has received extensive training in nutritional medicine.

If you would like more
information about natural and
divine healing, or information about
Divine Health Nutritional Products,
you may contact Dr. Colbert at:

DR. DON COLBERT
1908 Boothe Circle
Longwood, FL 32750
Telephone: 407–331–7007
(For ordering products only)
Dr. Colbert's Web site is
www.drcolbert.com.

Disclaimer: Dr. Colbert and the staff of Divine Health Wellness Center are prohibited from addressing a patient's medical condition by phone, facsimile or e-mail. Please refer questions related to your medical condition to your own primary care physician.